HYPERB[...]
STRETCHING [...]
FOR SENIORS

Unlock Flexibility and Mobility at Any Age

William G. Buchanan

TABLE OF CONTENT

INTRODUCTION

Hyperbolic Stretching Exercise for Seniors is an informative guide on how to enhance the flexibility and mobility of seniors through the use of targeted stretching exercises. This book will be of great interest to anyone who is interested in improving their overall physical health and well-being, especially those over the age of sixty. It is designed to help seniors maintain and improve the flexibility, range of motion, and balance in their bodies. It focuses on stretching and strengthening exercises which can help improve posture, reduce the risk of falls, and decrease the risk of injury. The book covers a wide range of topics, from basic stretching exercises to advanced flexibility training. It also provides information on injury prevention, risk factors, and important safety tips. This book is a must-read for seniors who want to take control of their physical health and move to a healthier lifestyle.

Hyperbolic Stretching Exercise for Seniors is written in an easy-to-understand manner and is backed by medical research and studies. It covers a wide range of topics, such as the benefits of stretching, proper form and technique for each exercise, and the importance of warming up and cooling down. It also provides detailed instructions on how to safely complete each exercise, as well as recommendations for rest periods between sets. The book also includes helpful tips and tricks on how to maximize results and stay motivated. For those who are just starting out, or for those who are more experienced, this book is a great resource for learning how to properly and safely stretch and strengthen the body.

CHAPTER ONE

Benefits of Hyperbolic Stretching Exercise for Seniors

Hyperbolic stretching exercise for seniors is a great way to improve flexibility, strength, posture, and overall well-being. This type of stretching is a combination of static, dynamic, and ballistic stretches. Hyperbolic stretching is an effective way to increase your range of motion, reduce pain, and improve overall health.

Hyperbolic stretching is especially beneficial for seniors because it can help reduce the risk of falls and injuries. This type of stretching helps to reduce muscle tension, increase flexibility, and improve posture. It is important to remember that seniors should always stretch properly and under the guidance of a qualified professional.

There are several benefits to hyperbolic stretching exercises for seniors. It can increase joint mobility, improve posture and balance, and reduce the risk of injury. Additionally, it can improve coordination, enhance muscular strength and endurance, and reduce stiffness and soreness in the muscles.

Hyperbolic stretching can also help to improve circulation and reduce inflammation in the joints. Improved circulation helps to carry oxygen and nutrients to the tissues, which can help to reduce pain and improve overall health. In addition, increased flexibility and range of motion can help seniors perform everyday tasks with ease.

Furthermore, hyperbolic stretching can help to reduce stress and tension. This type of stretching helps to relax the muscles, which can help to reduce stress and improve mental clarity. It can also help to improve mood and relieve anxiety.

Finally, hyperbolic stretching can be a great way for seniors to stay fit and healthy. It can help to improve physical fitness and cardiovascular health, as well as increase muscle tone. Additionally, it can help to improve balance, coordination, and agility.

In conclusion, hyperbolic stretching exercise for seniors is a great way to improve flexibility, strength, posture, and overall well-being. It can help to reduce the risk of injury, improve circulation, and reduce stress and tension. Additionally, it can help to increase joint mobility and improve physical fitness. For seniors, hyperbolic stretching can be an excellent way to stay fit and healthy.

Improved Flexibility and Mobility

As we age, our flexibility and mobility can become severely limited due to a number of factors, including muscle and joint stiffness, decreased range of motion, and reduced strength and coordination. Fortunately, seniors can benefit from engaging in hyperbolic stretching exercises. Hyperbolic stretching is a type of dynamic stretching that combines stretching and strength-building exercises to improve flexibility and mobility.

Hyperbolic stretching exercises involve stretching the body in a variety of directions and ranges of motion. This type of dynamic stretching helps to increase range of motion, improve coordination, and increase muscle strength. As a result, seniors can find it easier to perform everyday activities such as walking, bending, and reaching.

In addition to increasing flexibility and mobility, hyperbolic stretching exercises can also improve balance and posture. By strengthening the muscles and stretching the joints, hyperbolic stretching exercises can help to correct posture and improve balance. This is especially beneficial for seniors, as poor balance and posture can lead to falls and other dangerous accidents.

Hyperbolic stretching exercises can also help to improve overall health and well-being. By increasing flexibility and mobility, seniors can reduce the risk of injury and reduce pain in the joints. In addition, hyperbolic stretching exercises can help to improve circulation, which can help to reduce fatigue and improve energy levels.

In conclusion, hyperbolic stretching exercises can be beneficial for seniors in a number of ways. By increasing flexibility and mobility, improving balance and posture, and improving overall health and well-being, hyperbolic stretching exercises can help seniors to remain active and independent for longer.

Improved Balance and Posture

It is no secret that physical activity can bring a variety of health benefits to seniors, including improved balance and posture. Hyperbolic stretching exercises are a great way for seniors to improve their balance and posture and enjoy a variety of other health benefits.

Hyperbolic stretching is a series of stretching exercises designed to increase flexibility, strength, and mobility. This type of stretching targets specific muscle groups and helps to improve the range of motion in the joints. Additionally, hyperbolic stretching exercises can help to reduce tension and pain in the muscles and joints, as well as improve balance and posture.

One of the primary benefits of hyperbolic stretching for seniors is improved balance and posture. Improved balance and posture can help to reduce the risk of falls, which can be especially important for seniors who are at a higher risk of falling. Hyperbolic stretching can also help to improve coordination, which can help seniors to better navigate their environment and remain independent.

In addition to improved balance and posture, seniors can also benefit from hyperbolic stretching in other ways. Regular stretching can help to improve circulation and reduce stiffness in the joints, which can help to improve mobility and reduce the risk of injury. Additionally, hyperbolic stretching can help to improve muscle tone and strength, which can help to improve stability and reduce the risk of falls.

Overall, hyperbolic stretching exercises can be a great way for seniors to improve their balance and posture and enjoy a variety of other health benefits. Regular stretching can help to improve flexibility, strength, and mobility and reduce the risk of falls. Additionally, hyperbolic stretching can help to improve circulation and reduce stiffness in the joints, which can help to improve mobility and reduce the risk of injury. Improved balance and posture can also help seniors to better navigate their environment and remain independent.

For seniors looking to improve their balance and posture, hyperbolic stretching is an ideal exercise.

Not only can it help to reduce the risk of falls, but it can also help to improve strength, flexibility, and mobility, as well as reduce stiffness in the joints. With all of these benefits, it is no wonder why hyperbolic stretching is such a popular exercise for seniors.

Improved Coordination and Strength

Hyperbolic stretching exercise is a type of stretching regimen that has been found to be effective in a number of ways, particularly for seniors. This type of exercise helps to improve coordination, strength, and flexibility while also reducing the risk of injury.

Improved coordination is one of the major benefits of hyperbolic stretching exercise for seniors. Regular stretching helps to improve coordination by increasing the range of motion in the joints, as well as by increasing the amount of time it takes for the brain to send signals to the muscles. This improved coordination can help seniors to move more freely and with less risk of injury.

Strength is another benefit of hyperbolic stretching exercise for seniors. The stretching exercises help to strengthen the muscles, which can be particularly beneficial for seniors who may have lost some muscle mass due to age or inactivity. The stretching exercises also help to increase the range of motion of the muscles, which can help to reduce the risk of injury.

Hyperbolic stretching exercise can also improve flexibility. Stretching exercises help to improve flexibility by increasing the range of motion in the joints, as well as by helping to relax the muscles. This improved flexibility can help seniors move more easily and can reduce the risk of injury. Finally, hyperbolic stretching exercise can help to reduce the risk of injury. By increasing the range of motion in the joints, as well as by increasing the amount of time it takes for the brain to send signals to the muscles, the risk of injury is reduced. This is particularly beneficial for seniors who may be more prone to injury due to age or inactivity.

In conclusion, hyperbolic stretching exercise has a number of benefits for seniors, including improved coordination, strength, flexibility, and reduced risk of injury. Seniors who are looking to improve their health and fitness should consider adding this type of exercise to their routine.

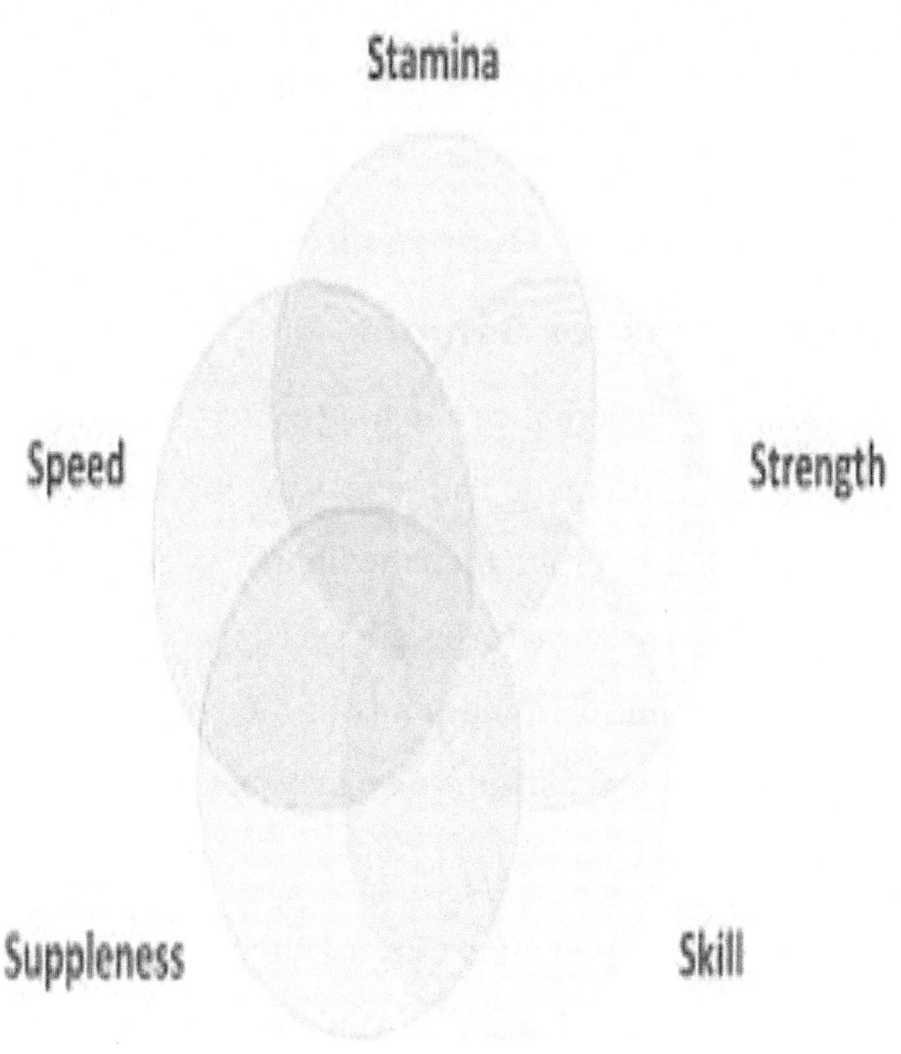

Stamina

Speed

Strength

Suppleness

Skill

Improved Coordination and Strength

CHAPTER TWO

Types of Hyperbolic Stretching Exercises for Seniors

Hyperbolic stretching exercises can be an efficient and safe way for seniors to improve their flexibility, strength, and mobility. These exercises are specially designed to target the muscles and joints of the body, making them suitable for seniors who may have age-related physical limitations.

Hyperbolic stretching is a form of dynamic stretching, which uses movements that gradually increase muscle tension, rather than static stretching which involves holding a single position for a period of time. This type of stretching is beneficial for seniors as it helps to improve their range of motion and flexibility. It also helps to reduce the risk of injury, as the muscles become more elastic and responsive.

There are many different types of hyperbolic stretching exercises that can be used to target different areas of the body. For example, hip flexor stretches can be used to target the hip flexors, which are responsible for helping to move the legs and hips. To perform this type of stretch, the person should stand with one foot in front of the other, and then slowly bend their front knee and push their hips forward. This movement should be repeated several times on both sides.

Other types of hyperbolic stretching exercises include shoulder stretches, back bends, and leg stretches. Shoulder stretches are beneficial for seniors as they help to increase the range of motion in the shoulder joint and reduce stiffness in the muscles. Back bends can help improve posture, while leg stretches can help to strengthen the muscles of the lower body.

It is important for seniors to perform these exercises properly in order to get the most benefit from them. It is best to start with short, slow stretches and gradually increase the intensity as the person becomes more comfortable with the movements. It is also important to make sure that the person is not overexerting themselves, as this can lead to injury.

Overall, hyperbolic stretching exercises can be an effective way for seniors to improve their flexibility, strength, and mobility. These exercises should be done slowly and with proper form in order to avoid injury. With proper execution, hyperbolic stretching exercises can be a great way for seniors to keep fit and improve their overall well-being.

Standing Exercises

Standing exercises are a type of hyperbolic stretching exercise that many seniors can benefit from. Hyperbolic stretching is a form of stretching that uses specific body positions and postures to target the muscles and surrounding connective tissues. This type of stretching helps to improve flexibility, strength, and range of motion. The exercises can be done while standing, lying down, or sitting.

For seniors, standing exercises are a great way to improve their general mobility. They can help to reduce pain in the joints, muscles, and other soft tissues. Standing exercises can also help to improve balance and stability. This is especially important for seniors as it can help to prevent trips and falls.

The key to getting the most benefit from standing exercises is to make sure the exercise is performed correctly. It is important to focus on proper form and breathing techniques to ensure the exercises are done safely and effectively. It is also important to avoid overexerting oneself and to take plenty of breaks if the exercises become too difficult.

When performing standing exercises, it is important to choose the appropriate level of intensity and range of motion. For seniors, it is best to start with basic exercises and gradually increase the difficulty as they become more comfortable with the movements. It is also important to focus on maintaining proper form throughout the exercise.

In addition to improving mobility, standing exercises can also help to improve overall health and well-being. This is because the exercises can help to increase circulation and stimulate the release of endorphins. This can lead to a feeling of increased energy and improved mood.

Overall, standing exercises are a great way for seniors to improve their flexibility, strength, and balance. By focusing on proper form and intensity, seniors can get the most benefit from these exercises while also avoiding injury. By doing these exercises regularly, seniors can enjoy improved mobility, increased energy, and better overall health.

Seated Exercises

Seated exercises are a type of hyperbolic stretching exercise specifically tailored for seniors. These exercises can help improve flexibility, strength, and balance while reducing the risk of injury. The benefits of seated exercises can be especially beneficial for seniors who may not be able to engage in more strenuous physical activities due to age or physical limitations.

Seated exercises are designed to be low-impact, making them suitable for those with joint pain, limited mobility, or other physical conditions. They can help improve range of motion, balance, and coordination. Seated exercises can be done in a variety of ways, such as sitting in a chair or on the floor. They can also include a variety of stretches, such as seated forward folds, seated side stretches, and seated spinal twists.

These exercises can be done at home with minimal equipment, making them an accessible and cost-effective form of exercise. Seated exercises can also help improve posture, circulation, and breathing. In addition, they can help reduce stress and tension, as well as improve mental clarity and focus.

Seated exercises can be particularly beneficial for seniors who may have difficulty with standing exercises due to balance issues or joint pain. This form of exercise can also help reduce the risk of falls, as it can help improve balance and coordination.

Overall, seated exercises are an excellent form of exercise for seniors. They can help improve flexibility, strength, and balance while reducing the risk of injury. They can also help improve posture, circulation, and breathing while reducing stress and tension. For seniors who may have difficulty with standing exercises, seated exercises can help reduce the risk of falls while still providing the same benefits.

Seated exercises can be done at home with minimal equipment, making them an accessible and cost-effective form of exercise for seniors. For those looking to get started, it's important to consult with a physician or physical therapist to determine the best exercises for their needs and abilities.

Floor Exercises

Floor exercises are an essential part of hyperbolic stretching for seniors. These exercises involve stretches that target the entire body, from the feet to the head. Not only do floor exercises offer the benefit of increased flexibility and strength, but they can also help seniors improve their balance and coordination.

Floor exercises are typically performed on a mat or other soft surface. Before beginning any stretching routine, it is important to warm up the body. This can be done by doing a few minutes of light aerobic activity, such as walking or jogging. Once the body is warm, seniors can begin the stretches.

The most basic floor exercises involve stretching the major muscle groups. For example, a senior can lie on their back and extend their arms above their head. They can then reach out to each side, feeling the stretch in their chest, shoulders, and arms. To add resistance, they can hold a light weight or stretch band in each hand and use it to pull their arms back.

Other floor exercises involve more complex movements. For example, a senior may use a foam roller to roll out tight muscles in their back, neck, and shoulders. They can also do a variety of leg stretches, such as lying on their back and lifting one leg at a time into the air.

Floor exercises are a great way for seniors to stay flexible and strong. They can also help improve balance and coordination, which can help prevent falls. Additionally, floor exercises can help to reduce stress and improve overall wellbeing. With regular practice, these exercises can help seniors remain active and independent for years to come.

In short, floor exercises are an important part of hyperbolic stretching for seniors. They can help to improve flexibility, strength, balance, and coordination. Additionally, these exercises can help to reduce stress and improve overall wellbeing. With regular practice, floor exercises can help seniors remain active and independent for years to come.

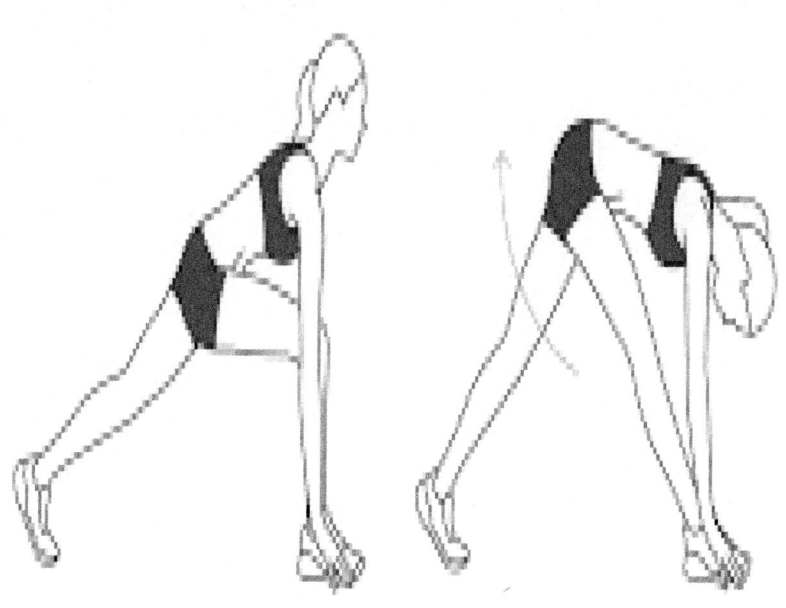

Floor Exercise

CHAPTER THREE

Safety and Precautions for Hyperbolic Stretching Exercise for Senior

Stretching techniques like hyperbolic stretching are intended to promote flexibility, enhance posture, and lower the chance of injury. All ages may benefit from these exercises, although seniors may need to take particular care while doing them.

Seniors need to be aware that hyperbolic stretching might be more demanding than conventional stretching. It's crucial to start off gently and progressively increase the stretching's intensity over time. In order to prevent damage, it's crucial to make sure the workouts are done properly. Seniors who are new to hyperbolic stretching should seek the advice of a certified teacher to make sure the exercises are done properly and securely.

Seniors should drink plenty of water both before and after stretching since dehydration may cause weariness and disorientation. Moreover, stretching should be done after a complete warm-up and cool-down. Light aerobic workouts like walking or running should be included in the warm-up routine. Light stretching should be done as a cool-down after stretching.

Seniors should be aware that hyperbolic stretching may be more painful or uncomfortable than ordinary stretching since it is more vigorous. Seniors should cease stretching as soon as they experience any pain or discomfort and get professional advice. Seniors should also see a doctor before starting any stretching program since the severity of hyperbolic stretching may make certain medical issues worse.

Seniors should also be aware that if hyperbolic stretching is done incorrectly, it may be harmful. Following a skilled instructor's instructions is crucial since using poor form might result in harm. Seniors should also refrain from stretching until they are completely exhausted since doing so might be dangerous.

In conclusion, older citizens may benefit from hyperbolic stretching exercises, but it's crucial to practice care and safety. Seniors should begin their activities softly and build up to a higher level of intensity over time. Before and after stretching, students should make sure they are well hydrated and warmed up. They should also obtain medical counsel before starting any stretching routine and refrain from stretching until they get exhausted. Lastly, to ensure that the exercises are carried out safely and properly, seniors should always adhere to the directions of a certified teacher.

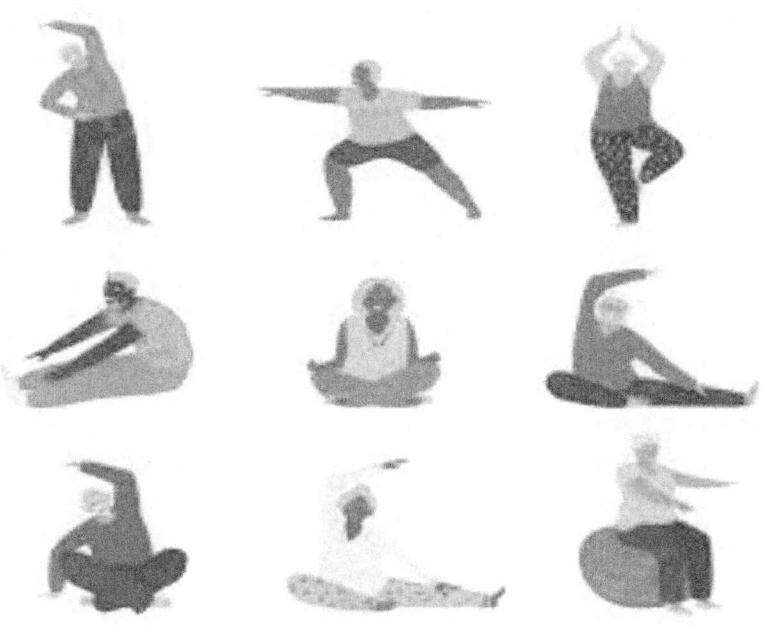

Stretching Exercises for Seniors

CONCLUSION

Finally, hyperbolic stretching exercises might be a great approach for elders to maintain their health and physical activity. The stretching exercises may be modified to meet the person's current level of fitness and are personalized to the person's demands. The workouts may aid in lowering the chance of injury since they are designed to be both safe and efficient. Also, they may aid in enhancing coordination, balance, and flexibility. Exercises for hyperbolic stretching are simple to add into your regular routine and may be performed at home or under supervision. In the end, they provide seniors with a range of advantages that may assist to enhance their general health and wellbeing. While there isn't a single fitness regimen that works for everyone, hyperbolic stretching is a great choice for seniors who want to maintain an active lifestyle.

Exercises that include hyperbolic stretching might assist seniors in maintaining their physical health, but it's crucial to keep in mind that mental wellness is just as important. Stretching may promote calmness and relaxation as well as stress relief. Also, it may aid in enhancing cognitive abilities and lowering the danger of cognitive decline. Finding a balance between physical and mental health is crucial for seniors in order to preserve overall wellness.

In the end, hyperbolic stretching may be a great approach for older people to keep fit and active. Always get medical advice before beginning any new fitness program, and make sure the workouts are suited to the individual's requirements. Seniors may benefit from hyperbolic stretching exercises and experience better physical and mental health with the correct direction and commitment.